MW01104948

RESET:

breathe

JOURNAL

TRACEY GAIRNS BRIOUX

I would like to dedicate this journal to the RESET:breathe community. You are beautiful, strong and brave people who have taught me the true power of community. I am so grateful for you.

I would also like to dedicate this to two beautiful angels - Belinda and Anna. You positively impacted all who knew you. Thank you for the lessons you have left on this earth.

Printed in Canada

Hi there! Welcome to the RESET:breathe journal and thank you for choosing this book as a tool to create more peace in your life. I am so glad you are here!

My name is Tracey Gairns Brioux and I am the owner/founder of RESET:breathe. I created this community in 2017 when the youngest of my four kids was about to turn one. It wasn't because I was a mom of four who had so much time on her hands that she thought she would throw a business in the mix, it was because I literally had reached my breaking point and I just needed to do something about it.

My thirties brought me a lot of lessons. The biggest ones unfortunately came from loss. When I was 30, I lost a baby at four months pregnant and a few years later I lost my really close friend, Belinda "B," to cancer who was only 33. We all experience loss at some point in our lives but these experiences woke something inside me that I find hard to explain. Watching my friend fight so hard JUST to be here and live for her baby boy is something I can't put into words. It was devastating, tragic and inspiring. It changed me forever.

When my son was born a few years later, we almost lost him too. The months following, I was just hanging on as we visited doctor after doctor and had test after test. I was just so freaking tired and felt so lost. He is a miracle boy and I'm so happy to say he's doing incredible but his first year brought me to that breaking point I mentioned. I had to do something to improve my life. I had to do something to better the lives of other women and men who were struggling too. Losing my friend taught me what a gift life is to get to live it. Almost losing my son reminded me we need to love living it.

In large part because of my parents, I have been active my whole life. I started teaching Pilates and fitness in my 20s and well- I just finished my thirties. I don't always love to exercise but I will never stop because of the peace that it gives my mind and the energy it gives my body. Through everything hard I have been through, moving my body has saved my life. I have sweated out so much stress and literally cried during many runs and every single time, I came home feeling better. I have taught thousands of classes and have never ever, ever met anyone who regretted showing up and moving when it was done. It's an immediate guarantee to feel better and that's why I keep at it and why I'm so inspired watching others doing it. It's truly so awesome to be around the energy of someone who just moved their body.

I love seeing people make positive changes in their lives. I actually cry about it on a regular basis (I'm a crier). Something that keeps me up at night though is watching women start, feel better, feel happier, feel more energized and then give up when life gets in the way. It sucks to watch that. As a society, we have glorified busyness. We have glorified hard work = high performance. We have made the woman who does it all for everyone the standard to strive for. In doing that, we have also created a very tired and worn out culture where women slide themselves down the priority list because everything else feels more important and well, we just can't disappoint. It's time to shift that.

The devastations I experienced above were just two of the hard life lessons that taught me there is nothing more important than your health. One of my favourite quotes is "when you have your health you have 1000 dreams, when you don't, you have one." I think of my friend B everytime I read that. I remember her energy and her smile and her vibrancy most, but I also haven't forgotten the look in her eyes when all she wanted was to just live and be well.

As a trainer, I have watched the start then stop pattern many times. It makes me so sad. I don't believe women give up on movement because they are lazy, which I know is what they tell themselves, I believe it's actually the exact opposite. I believe women give up on it because deep down they feel everything else should come first. Guilt— I wish I could eliminate it off of this earth. I don't think I have ever met a woman who hasn't or doesn't experience it regularly. I remember one time I asked my husband if he ever feels guilty when he leaves the kids to go to work and he looked at me with complete wonder and said simply "no." Okay then (insert eyeroll emoji), I guess that's just me. Now, let's get to you.

You right here. You reading this right now are so important. You are such a beautiful human and you bring so much light into this world. Don't say "not me." Stop it. I know how you think but seriously, you do. You are so awesome! If you are struggling to believe that today, think of your little face when you were a child. Imagine looking in their eyes and not believing that little person wasn't awesome?! You were then and you are now. You deserve to show up every day feeling the best you absolutely can. Even if you were up all night with a baby who needs you and you are so tired you forget your name and what you bought online when you were half asleep, you still deserve time to feel better.

Thirty minutes is just 2% of your day. We all deserve that as a minimum but when you start to carve that time out fresh, it can be overwhelming. In all the years I have been doing this, I have seen that what really works is small steps. Slowly integrating little changes into your life so that when you stick with them, they change your life. Not exercising right now? Don't go all out for seven days straight. Make a goal to do ten minutes a day, or two, 30-minute workouts per week. It's just enough to create a difference but not so much that when life happens, like your dog gets sick or work gets crazy, that you feel it's too much and stop. I promise you, the small changes add up and that's where true growth happens.

The RESET:breathe journal is a compilation of all things 'feel good.' Everyone was born with the right to live their life feeling the best they absolutely can but sometimes we just forget how. Each day you will be asked to track the things that contribute to us feeling our best. You can pick what to start with and please don't feel discouraged by picking just one thing. This is not a one size fits all; it's meant to simply be your guide and you do what feels right for you. Focus on the things that make YOU feel a little better each day. Not all days are great days but every day has good in it and we will find it here.

The daily prompts will always include a space for you to track your sleep, your energy, your movement, your water intake and your greens. I chose these things because they ALL impact our energy and vitality. Sleep is so underrated and it affects everything you do. It doesn't mean every night has to be a great night's sleep (it won't be; 11 years into parenting and my kids still don't sleep through the night); it's intended to be a teaching tool. Being up all night affects your energy. Only getting four hours of sleep doesn't help us manage 3 pm very well. Your energy affects your mood and motivation which in turn can affect whether you move your body, how well you eat and how much water you drink. I know the drill....tired...drink coffee...forget water. When I get more rest, I have more energy to move, I drink more water and my energy levels are best. Can't possibly get a good night's sleep right now because of your kids? Learn to nap or sit down and do nothing!! It's amazing!! I have napped under a pile of unfolded laundry before and I'm not a bit shy to admit it!!

Greens are something I encourage everyone to "add" into their routine. There are days I eat really well and there are days I don't— my rule of thumb is I try to eat greens every day. You don't need to remove anything but you can add this in and it's always good for you.

Instead of asking you to write down the same things every day, I chose some of my favourite feel-goods and will alternate them every five days. A couple of these feel-goods are gratitude and affirmations. Practicing gratitude is so important, especially when life feels hard. It doesn't mean we don't acknowledge the hard stuff, not at all; it means that we train our minds to never stop looking for the good stuff. I have watched many of my reset community members go through really hard things. When they would show up during those hard times, they almost always shared how grateful they were for their ability to move. It was a tool they used to help them get through it and they recognized that. Sometimes hanging on to those little things, or reminding yourself of something that made you smile is what can really carry us through the big storms. Honestly, watching people like that is the most inspiring part of my job. Back to the journal.

Affirmations are something I started about a year into RESET:breathe at the end of each class. I felt really weird and awkward doing them at first but it was only because I had spent years mastering negative self-talk. It was eye-opening to me to see how uncomfortable talking positively to myself was/ is and that is why we need to do it more and why I'm asking you to do it there. We need to get over it. Tim Ferriss says "the most important actions are never comfortable." I promise you, changing the way you think about yourself can change your life. Affirmations are often "I am" statements. Like "I am strong," "I am resilient," etc. but they can also be anything where you are speaking about yourself positively: "I can do hard things" (one of my faves), "I protect my family," "I give love to those around me." You can choose what words resonate with you. This is a guide and I want you to make it fit what you need. Just remember the point is to be kind to yourself.

Each day you will be asked to write down two priorities. These are your two most important non-negotiables for your health and well being, the things that for you will make the biggest impact. Sometimes that might be exercise, it might be a nap, it might be cleaning out your car or it might be working on your new website. Try to keep things like framing pictures or wrapping presents off this list; here is where you want the most important things that will make you feel good after. Think quality not quantity and that's why we are only choosing two. We want to do less things that create more peace.

This leads me to the items that say "I release" and "where can I save energy?" These are so important. We are not meant to do and accomplish all the things without help. I highly encourage you to ask for more of it. This is a really hard one for a lot of people but it's incredibly important. What can you take off your to do list? What is taking up space and energy that you can get help with? Is it really that important? What is something you are worrying about that you can let go of? If you are an empath like me, you likely carry a lot of stuff. Here is where I want you to acknowledge it and then release it. For example, "today I release that my kids went to school with mismatched socks" (mine rarely do), or "I release the hard stuff I saw on the news." Your energy is so valuable; here is where you focus on protecting it.

The additional prompts are to focus on celebrating wins big or small and overcoming hard things. They don't need to be huge like getting a promotion or winning the lottery—although definitely write that down if it happens, it can be things like "today I let myself take a rest," or "I kept my patience when my kids were losing it because I wouldn't buy them Timbits." Find your wins. Celebrate them!

Lastly, I don't want you to ever stop dreaming. I don't want you to ever stop setting goals for yourself. It's proven that when we write our goals and dreams down, when we put them out there, they are more likely to come true. You are never too old to stop dreaming. I also ask that when you do this, you take a minute and visualize what it will feel like when these goals and dreams come true. I have a dream of one day taking my family to Australia. I have replayed the feeling of us all getting off the plane together so many times and how proud I will feel when it comes true. I try and keep that energy with me as often as I can. Envision the version of you who has reached those goals and dreams.

As a society that is collectively very hard on ourselves, we need to change how we think and treat ourselves. Get through your first week of reading before bed or do it for the first time?! Write that down!! Make your first green smoothie and half like it?! Write that down!! Make it through bedtime without yelling?? WRITE THAT DOWN!! I know I said this already but I will shout this from the rooftops if you give me a ladder: it's the little things that count. It's the little things that add up. It's the little things that are done consistently over time, that make the greatest difference. Remember when you were little and took your first step?? Ok, maybe not, but you were there once and you definitely got back up after you fell. Remember learning to read, swim, ride a bike or tie your shoe? These weren't easy, but you kept going. Just because you are grown doesn't mean you still can't create growth, love and happiness in your life. A wise friend and mentor of mine told me once, the greatest obstacle you will ever face in your life, is yourself. #truth

YOU'VE GOT THIS!!

At the back of the journal, I created challenges for you to do throughout your time here. You can do them more than once. You can do the same one over and over. I also included a few pages for you to just write. If you have a lot on your mind, dreams, goals or something happy you want to take note of, this is the space for that.

I hope your journey with this journal is a positive one. I hope it helps you learn to truly love the beautiful person you are and allows your light to shine even brighter. I hope through this work, you will find it easier to celebrate your wins, celebrate your strengths and be proud of your strides forward, both big and small.

You are amazing. You are awesome and once again- I'm SO glad you are here!

Sending you so much love,

xoxo, Tracey

DATE_____

SLEEP: ☐ 3-5hours   ☐ 5-6hours   ☐ 7+hours

WATER: ⬚⬚⬚⬚⬚⬚⬚ GREENS: _____

MOVEMENT: _____ ENERGY: _____

PRIORITIES FOR TODAY:

1. _____

2. _____

TODAY I AM GRATEFUL FOR:

1. _____

_____

2. _____

_____

3. _____

_____

AFFIRMATION: _____

_____

_____

_____

_____

_____

_____

_____

_____

"Turn your wounds into wisdom." —Oprah Winfrey

DATE_____

SLEEP: ☐ 3-5hours ☐ 5-6hours ☐ 7+hours

WATER: ☐☐☐☐☐☐☐☐ GREENS: _____

MOVEMENT: _____ ENERGY: _____

PRIORITIES FOR TODAY:

1. _____

2. _____

MY WINS:

1. _____

_____

2. _____

_____

3. _____

_____

WHERE CAN I SAVE ENERGY TODAY? _____

_____

_____

_____

_____

_____

_____

_____

_____

"I am resilient and strong."

DATE_____

SLEEP: ☐ 3-5hours ☐ 5-6hours ☐ 7+hours

WATER: ☐ ☐ ☐ ☐ ☐ ☐ ☐ GREENS: _____

MOVEMENT: _____ ENERGY: _____

PRIORITIES FOR TODAY:

1. _____

2. _____

I FELT MY BEST TODAY WHEN: _____

_____

_____

_____

_____

_____

_____

ONE GOAL I AM WORKING ON:_____

_____

_____

_____

_____

_____

_____

"Reach change, enduring change, happens one step at a time."
—Ruth Bader Ginsburg

DATE_____

SLEEP: ☐ 3-5hours ☐ 5-6hours ☐ 7+hours

WATER: ☐☐☐☐☐☐☐ GREENS: _____

MOVEMENT: _____ ENERGY: _____

PRIORITIES FOR TODAY:

1. _____

2. _____

TODAY I SMILED BECAUSE: _____

_____

_____

_____

_____

_____

_____

_____

ONE HARD THING I DID TODAY (OR YESTERDAY): _____

_____

_____

_____

_____

_____

_____

"It is never too late to be what you might have been." —George Eliot

DATE_____

SLEEP: ☐ 3-5hours ☐ 5-6hours ☐ 7+hours

WATER: ☐☐☐☐☐☐☐☐ GREENS: _____

MOVEMENT: _____ ENERGY: _____

PRIORITIES FOR TODAY:

1. _____

2. _____

TODAY I LET GO OF: _____

_____

_____

_____

_____

_____

_____

_____

ONE DREAM I AM WORKING ON: _____

_____

_____

_____

_____

_____

_____

_____

"We are who we believe we are." —C.S Lewis

DATE_____

SLEEP: ☐ 3-5hours ☐ 5-6hours ☐ 7+hours

WATER: ☐☐☐☐☐☐☐ GREENS: _____

MOVEMENT: _____ ENERGY: _____

PRIORITIES FOR TODAY:

1. _____

2. _____

TODAY I AM GRATEFUL FOR:

1. _____
_____

2. _____
_____

3. _____
_____

AFFIRMATION: _____
_____
_____
_____
_____
_____
_____
_____

"I can do hard things."

DATE_____

SLEEP: ☐ 3-5hours ☐ 5-6hours ☐ 7+hours

WATER: ☐☐☐☐☐☐☐ GREENS: _____

MOVEMENT: _____ ENERGY: _____

PRIORITIES FOR TODAY:

1. _____

2. _____

MY WINS:

1. _____

_____

2. _____

_____

3. _____

_____

WHERE CAN I SAVE ENERGY TODAY? _____

_____

_____

_____

_____

_____

_____

_____

_____

*"When we have our health we hae 1000 dreams,
when we don't, we have one."* —Unknown

DATE_____

SLEEP: ☐ 3-5hours ☐ 5-6hours ☐ 7+hours

WATER: ☐☐☐☐☐☐☐ GREENS: _____

MOVEMENT: _____ ENERGY: _____

PRIORITIES FOR TODAY:

1. _____

2. _____

I FELT MY BEST TODAY WHEN: _____

_____

_____

_____

_____

_____

_____

ONE GOAL I AM WORKING ON:_____

_____

_____

_____

_____

_____

_____

"I bring light into the lives of the people I love."

DATE_____

SLEEP: ☐ 3-5hours ☐ 5-6hours ☐ 7+hours

WATER: ☐ ☐ ☐ ☐ ☐ ☐ ☐ GREENS: _____

MOVEMENT: _____ ENERGY: _____

PRIORITIES FOR TODAY:

1. _____

2. _____

TODAY I SMILED BECAUSE: _____

_____

_____

_____

_____

_____

_____

ONE HARD THING I DID TODAY (OR YESTERDAY): _____

_____

_____

_____

_____

_____

_____

"Be courageous and live the life that your heart is guiding you toward."
—Bronnie Ware

DATE_____

SLEEP: ☐ 3-5hours ☐ 5-6hours ☐ 7+hours

WATER: ⬛⬛⬛⬛⬛⬛⬛ GREENS: _____

MOVEMENT: _____ ENERGY: _____

PRIORITIES FOR TODAY:

1. _____

2. _____

TODAY I LET GO OF: _____

_____

_____

_____

_____

_____

_____

ONE DREAM I AM WORKING ON: _____

_____

_____

_____

_____

_____

_____

"One day you will look back and see that all along, you were blooming."
—Morgan Harper Nichols

DATE _____

SLEEP: ☐ 3-5hours ☐ 5-6hours ☐ 7+hours

WATER: ☐ ☐ ☐ ☐ ☐ ☐ ☐ GREENS: _____

MOVEMENT: _____ ENERGY: _____

PRIORITIES FOR TODAY:

1. _____

2. _____

TODAY I AM GRATEFUL FOR:

1. _____

_____

2. _____

_____

3. _____

_____

AFFIRMATION: _____

_____

_____

_____

_____

_____

_____

_____

_____

"You never have to ask anyone permission to lead."
—Kamala Harris

DATE_____

SLEEP: ☐ 3-5hours ☐ 5-6hours ☐ 7+hours

WATER: ☐☐☐☐☐☐☐ GREENS: _____

MOVEMENT: _____ ENERGY: _____

PRIORITIES FOR TODAY:

1. _____

2. _____

MY WINS:

1. _____

_____

2. _____

_____

3. _____

_____

WHERE CAN I SAVE ENERGY TODAY? _____

_____

_____

_____

_____

_____

_____

_____

"Great things are done by a series of small things brought together."
—Vincent Van Gogh

DATE_____

SLEEP: ☐ 3-5hours ☐ 5-6hours ☐ 7+hours

WATER: ☐☐☐☐☐☐☐ GREENS: _____

MOVEMENT: _____ ENERGY: _____

PRIORITIES FOR TODAY:

1. _____

2. _____

I FELT MY BEST TODAY WHEN: _____

_____

_____

_____

_____

_____

_____

_____

ONE GOAL I AM WORKING ON:_____

_____

_____

_____

_____

_____

_____

"And now that you don't have to be perfect, you can be good."
—John Steinbeck

DATE _____

SLEEP: ☐ 3-5hours ☐ 5-6hours ☐ 7+hours

WATER: ⊔⊔⊔⊔⊔⊔⊔⊔ GREENS: _____

MOVEMENT: _____ ENERGY: _____

PRIORITIES FOR TODAY:

1. _____

2. _____

TODAY I SMILED BECAUSE: _____

_____

_____

_____

_____

_____

_____

ONE HARD THING I DID TODAY (OR YESTERDAY): _____

_____

_____

_____

_____

_____

_____

_____

_____

*"You can't go back and change the beginning, but you can start
where you are and change the ending."* —C.S. Lewis

DATE_____

SLEEP: ☐ 3-5hours ☐ 5-6hours ☐ 7+hours

WATER: ☐☐☐☐☐☐☐ GREENS: _____

MOVEMENT: _____ ENERGY: _____

PRIORITIES FOR TODAY:

1. _____

2. _____

TODAY I LET GO OF: _____

_____

_____

_____

_____

_____

_____

ONE DREAM I AM WORKING ON: _____

_____

_____

_____

_____

_____

_____

"Imperfection is a form of freedom." —Anh Ngo

DATE_____

SLEEP: ☐ 3-5hours ☐ 5-6hours ☐ 7+hours

WATER: ☐☐☐☐☐☐☐ GREENS: _____

MOVEMENT: _____ ENERGY: _____

PRIORITIES FOR TODAY:

1. _____

2. _____

TODAY I AM GRATEFUL FOR:

1. _____
_____

2. _____
_____

3. _____
_____

AFFIRMATION: _____
_____
_____
_____
_____
_____
_____
_____

"The most effective way to do it, is to do it." —Amelia Earhart

DATE_____

SLEEP: ☐ 3-5hours ☐ 5-6hours ☐ 7+hours

WATER: ☐ ☐ ☐ ☐ ☐ ☐ ☐ GREENS: _____

MOVEMENT: _____ ENERGY: _____

PRIORITIES FOR TODAY:

1. _____

2. _____

MY WINS:

1. _____

_____

2. _____

_____

3. _____

_____

WHERE CAN I SAVE ENERGY TODAY? _____

_____

_____

_____

_____

_____

_____

_____

"The joy we feel has little to do with the circumstances of our lives and everything to do with the focus of our lives." —Russell M. Nelson

DATE_____

SLEEP: ☐ 3-5hours ☐ 5-6hours ☐ 7+hours

WATER: ☐☐☐☐☐☐☐ GREENS: _____

MOVEMENT: _____ ENERGY: _____

PRIORITIES FOR TODAY:

1. _____

2. _____

I FELT MY BEST TODAY WHEN: _____

_____

_____

_____

_____

_____

_____

_____

ONE GOAL I AM WORKING ON:_____

_____

_____

_____

_____

_____

_____

_____

"It takes courage to open ourselves up to joy." —Brene Brown

DATE_____

SLEEP: ☐ 3-5hours ☐ 5-6hours ☐ 7+hours

WATER: ☐☐☐☐☐☐☐ GREENS: _____

MOVEMENT: _____ ENERGY: _____

PRIORITIES FOR TODAY:

1. _____

2. _____

TODAY I SMILED BECAUSE: _____

_____

_____

_____

_____

_____

_____

_____

ONE HARD THING I DID TODAY (OR YESTERDAY): _____

_____

_____

_____

_____

_____

_____

_____

"It is not joy that makes us grateful, it is gratitude that makes us joyful." —Unknown

DATE_____

SLEEP: ☐ 3-5hours ☐ 5-6hours ☐ 7+hours

WATER: ☐☐☐☐☐☐☐ GREENS: _____

MOVEMENT: _____ ENERGY: _____

PRIORITIES FOR TODAY:

1. _____

2. _____

TODAY I LET GO OF: _____

_____

_____

_____

_____

_____

_____

ONE DREAM I AM WORKING ON: _____

_____

_____

_____

_____

_____

_____

_____

"You are the most valuable investment you will ever make." —Unknown

DATE _____

SLEEP: ☐ 3-5hours ☐ 5-6hours ☐ 7+hours

WATER: 🥛🥛🥛🥛🥛🥛🥛 GREENS: _____

MOVEMENT: _____ ENERGY: _____

PRIORITIES FOR TODAY:

1. _____

2. _____

TODAY I AM GRATEFUL FOR:

1. _____

_____

2. _____

_____

3. _____

_____

AFFIRMATION: _____

_____

_____

_____

_____

_____

_____

_____

"I showed up today and I am stronger for it."

DATE_____

SLEEP: ☐ 3-5hours ☐ 5-6hours ☐ 7+hours

WATER: ☐☐☐☐☐☐☐ GREENS: _____

MOVEMENT: _____ ENERGY: _____

PRIORITIES FOR TODAY:

1. _____

2. _____

MY WINS:

1. _____

_____

2. _____

_____

3. _____

_____

WHERE CAN I SAVE ENERGY TODAY? _____

_____

_____

_____

_____

_____

_____

_____

"Make happiness a priority and be gentle with yourself in the process."
—Bronnie Ware

DATE_____

SLEEP: ☐ 3-5hours ☐ 5-6hours ☐ 7+hours

WATER: ☐☐☐☐☐☐☐☐ GREENS: _____

MOVEMENT: _____ ENERGY: _____

PRIORITIES FOR TODAY:

1. _____

2. _____

I FELT MY BEST TODAY WHEN: _____

_____

_____

_____

_____

_____

_____

ONE GOAL I AM WORKING ON:_____

_____

_____

_____

_____

_____

_____

_____

"I let go of the outcome and let myself trust the process."
—Beautiful Mindset Life

DATE_____

SLEEP: ☐ 3-5hours ☐ 5-6hours ☐ 7+hours

WATER: ☐☐☐☐☐☐☐ GREENS: _____

MOVEMENT: _____ ENERGY: _____

PRIORITIES FOR TODAY:

1. _____

2. _____

TODAY I SMILED BECAUSE: _____

_____

_____

_____

_____

_____

_____

ONE HARD THING I DID TODAY (OR YESTERDAY): _____

_____

_____

_____

_____

_____

_____

_____

"I am worthy of a beautiful life."

DATE_____

SLEEP: ☐ 3-5hours ☐ 5-6hours ☐ 7+hours

WATER: ⊔⊔⊔⊔⊔⊔⊔ GREENS: _____

MOVEMENT: _____ ENERGY: _____

PRIORITIES FOR TODAY:

1. _____

2. _____

TODAY I LET GO OF: _____

_____

_____

_____

_____

_____

_____

ONE DREAM I AM WORKING ON: _____

_____

_____

_____

_____

_____

_____

"If you need something to satisfy your soul, let it be you this time."
—Beautiful Mindset Life

DATE_____

SLEEP: ☐ 3-5hours ☐ 5-6hours ☐ 7+hours

WATER: ☐☐☐☐☐☐☐☐ GREENS: _____

MOVEMENT: _____ ENERGY: _____

PRIORITIES FOR TODAY:

1. _____

2. _____

TODAY I AM GRATEFUL FOR:

1. _____

_____

2. _____

_____

3. _____

_____

AFFIRMATION: _____

_____

_____

_____

_____

_____

_____

_____

*"Self-care is sometimes just waking up, greeting the sun
and telling yourself this is your day." —Jennae Cecelia*

DATE_____

SLEEP: ☐ 3-5hours ☐ 5-6hours ☐ 7+hours

WATER: ☐☐☐☐☐☐☐ GREENS: _____

MOVEMENT: _____ ENERGY: _____

PRIORITIES FOR TODAY:

1. _____

2. _____

MY WINS:

1. _____

_____

2. _____

_____

3. _____

_____

WHERE CAN I SAVE ENERGY TODAY? _____

_____

_____

_____

_____

_____

_____

_____

"I am a warrior."

DATE_____

SLEEP: ☐ 3-5hours ☐ 5-6hours ☐ 7+hours

WATER: ☐☐☐☐☐☐☐ GREENS: _____

MOVEMENT: _____ ENERGY: _____

PRIORITIES FOR TODAY:

1. _____

2. _____

I FELT MY BEST TODAY WHEN: _____

_____

_____

_____

_____

_____

_____

_____

ONE GOAL I AM WORKING ON:_____

_____

_____

_____

_____

_____

_____

_____

"Flowers grow back even after the harshest winters, you will too."
—Jennae Cecelia

DATE_____

SLEEP: ☐ 3-5hours ☐ 5-6hours ☐ 7+hours

WATER: ☐☐☐☐☐☐☐☐ GREENS: _____

MOVEMENT: _____ ENERGY: _____

PRIORITIES FOR TODAY:

1. _____

2. _____

TODAY I SMILED BECAUSE: _____

_____

_____

_____

_____

_____

_____

_____

ONE HARD THING I DID TODAY (OR YESTERDAY): _____

_____

_____

_____

_____

_____

_____

_____

"Give thanks in everything." —1 Thess 5:18

DATE_____

SLEEP: ☐ 3-5hours ☐ 5-6hours ☐ 7+hours

WATER: ⊔⊔⊔⊔⊔⊔⊔⊔ GREENS: _____

MOVEMENT: _____ ENERGY: _____

PRIORITIES FOR TODAY:

1. _____

2. _____

TODAY I LET GO OF: _____

_____

_____

_____

_____

_____

_____

ONE DREAM I AM WORKING ON: _____

_____

_____

_____

_____

_____

_____

"I deserve the same love today as I did as a child. Infinite."

DATE_____

SLEEP: ☐ 3-5hours ☐ 5-6hours ☐ 7+hours

WATER: ☐☐☐☐☐☐☐☐ GREENS: _____

MOVEMENT: _____ ENERGY: _____

PRIORITIES FOR TODAY:

1. _____

2. _____

TODAY I AM GRATEFUL FOR:

1. _____
   _____

2. _____
   _____

3. _____
   _____

AFFIRMATION: _____
_____
_____
_____
_____
_____
_____
_____

"You can do anything but not everything." —Unknown

DATE_____

SLEEP: ☐ 3-5hours ☐ 5-6hours ☐ 7+hours

WATER: ☐☐☐☐☐☐☐☐ GREENS: _____

MOVEMENT: _____ ENERGY: _____

PRIORITIES FOR TODAY:

1. _____

2. _____

MY WINS:

1. _____

_____

2. _____

_____

3. _____

_____

WHERE CAN I SAVE ENERGY TODAY? _____

_____

_____

_____

_____

_____

_____

_____

"Give Grace." —Volume 18

DATE_____

SLEEP: ☐ 3-5hours ☐ 5-6hours ☐ 7+hours

WATER: ☐☐☐☐☐☐☐ GREENS: _____

MOVEMENT: _____ ENERGY: _____

PRIORITIES FOR TODAY:

1. _____

2. _____

I FELT MY BEST TODAY WHEN: _____

_____

_____

_____

_____

_____

_____

_____

ONE GOAL I AM WORKING ON:_____

_____

_____

_____

_____

_____

_____

_____

"Be bold and courageous. When you look back on your life, you'll regret the things you didn't do more than the ones you did." —H. Jackson Brown Jr.

DATE_____

SLEEP: ☐ 3-5hours ☐ 5-6hours ☐ 7+hours

WATER: ☐☐☐☐☐☐☐ GREENS: _____

MOVEMENT: _____ ENERGY: _____

PRIORITIES FOR TODAY:

1. _____

2. _____

TODAY I SMILED BECAUSE: _____

_____

_____

_____

_____

_____

_____

ONE HARD THING I DID TODAY (OR YESTERDAY): _____

_____

_____

_____

_____

_____

_____

_____

"When you undervalue what you do, the world will undervalue who you are."
—Oprah Winfrey

DATE_____

SLEEP: ☐ 3-5hours ☐ 5-6hours ☐ 7+hours

WATER: ⬡⬡⬡⬡⬡⬡⬡ GREENS: _____

MOVEMENT: _____ ENERGY: _____

PRIORITIES FOR TODAY:

1. _____

2. _____

TODAY I LET GO OF: _____

_____

_____

_____

_____

_____

_____

_____

ONE DREAM I AM WORKING ON: _____

_____

_____

_____

_____

_____

_____

_____

"I am the dreamer of my dreams. My dreams have no limits"

DATE_____

SLEEP: ☐ 3-5hours   ☐ 5-6hours   ☐ 7+hours

WATER: ☐☐☐☐☐☐☐   GREENS: _____

MOVEMENT: _____   ENERGY: _____

PRIORITIES FOR TODAY:

1. _____

2. _____

TODAY I AM GRATEFUL FOR:

1. _____

_____

2. _____

_____

3. _____

_____

AFFIRMATION: _____

_____

_____

_____

_____

_____

_____

_____

"My body is strong. My mind is peaceful. I am happy."

DATE_____

SLEEP: ☐ 3-5hours ☐ 5-6hours ☐ 7+hours

WATER: ☐☐☐☐☐☐☐☐ GREENS: _____

MOVEMENT: _____ ENERGY: _____

PRIORITIES FOR TODAY:

1. _____

2. _____

MY WINS:

1. _____
_____

2. _____
_____

3. _____
_____

WHERE CAN I SAVE ENERGY TODAY? _____
_____
_____
_____
_____
_____
_____
_____

*"True beauty is knowing who you are and what you want
and never apologizing for it."* —Pink

DATE_____

SLEEP: ☐ 3-5hours ☐ 5-6hours ☐ 7+hours

WATER: ☐☐☐☐☐☐☐ GREENS: _____

MOVEMENT: _____ ENERGY: _____

PRIORITIES FOR TODAY:

1. _____

2. _____

I FELT MY BEST TODAY WHEN: _____

_____

_____

_____

_____

_____

_____

ONE GOAL I AM WORKING ON:_____

_____

_____

_____

_____

_____

_____

"I am resilient and brave."

DATE_____

SLEEP: ☐ 3-5hours ☐ 5-6hours ☐ 7+hours

WATER: ☐☐☐☐☐☐☐ GREENS: _____

MOVEMENT: _____ ENERGY: _____

PRIORITIES FOR TODAY:

1. _____

2. _____

TODAY I SMILED BECAUSE: _____

_____

_____

_____

_____

_____

_____

_____

ONE HARD THING I DID TODAY (OR YESTERDAY): _____

_____

_____

_____

_____

_____

_____

_____

"A girl should be two things: Who and what she wants." —Coco Channel

DATE_____

SLEEP: ☐ 3-5hours ☐ 5-6hours ☐ 7+hours

WATER: ⊔⊔⊔⊔⊔⊔⊔ GREENS: _____

MOVEMENT: _____ ENERGY: _____

PRIORITIES FOR TODAY:

1. _____

2. _____

TODAY I LET GO OF: _____

_____

_____

_____

_____

_____

_____

_____

ONE DREAM I AM WORKING ON: _____

_____

_____

_____

_____

_____

_____

_____

*"Courage doesn't mean you don't get afraid. Courage means
you don't let fear stop you."* —Bethany Hamilton

DATE_____

SLEEP: ☐ 3-5hours   ☐ 5-6hours   ☐ 7+hours

WATER: ⊔⊔⊔⊔⊔⊔⊔   GREENS: _____

MOVEMENT: _____   ENERGY: _____

PRIORITIES FOR TODAY:

1. _____

2. _____

TODAY I AM GRATEFUL FOR:

1. _____

_____

2. _____

_____

3. _____

_____

AFFIRMATION: _____

_____

_____

_____

_____

_____

_____

_____

"I am unstoppable. I can do anything I sent my mind on."

DATE_____

SLEEP: ☐ 3-5hours ☐ 5-6hours ☐ 7+hours

WATER: ☐ ☐ ☐ ☐ ☐ ☐ ☐ GREENS: _____

MOVEMENT: _____ ENERGY: _____

PRIORITIES FOR TODAY:

1. _____

2. _____

MY WINS:

1. _____

_____

2. _____

_____

3. _____

_____

WHERE CAN I SAVE ENERGY TODAY? _____

_____

_____

_____

_____

_____

_____

_____

_____

"I am beautiful."

DATE_____

SLEEP: ☐ 3-5hours ☐ 5-6hours ☐ 7+hours

WATER: ☐ ☐ ☐ ☐ ☐ ☐ ☐ GREENS: _____

MOVEMENT: _____ ENERGY: _____

PRIORITIES FOR TODAY:

1. _____

2. _____

I FELT MY BEST TODAY WHEN: _____

_____

_____

_____

_____

_____

_____

ONE GOAL I AM WORKING ON:_____

_____

_____

_____

_____

_____

_____

"There is nothing stronger than a broken women who has rebuilt herself."
—Hannah Gadsby

DATE_____

SLEEP: ☐ 3-5hours ☐ 5-6hours ☐ 7+hours

WATER: ⊔⊔⊔⊔⊔⊔⊔ GREENS: _____

MOVEMENT: _____ ENERGY: _____

PRIORITIES FOR TODAY:

1. _____

2. _____

TODAY I SMILED BECAUSE: _____

_____

_____

_____

_____

_____

_____

_____

ONE HARD THING I DID TODAY (OR YESTERDAY): _____

_____

_____

_____

_____

_____

_____

_____

"Trust life a little bit." —Maya Angelou

DATE_____

SLEEP: ☐ 3-5hours ☐ 5-6hours ☐ 7+hours

WATER: ⊔⊔⊔⊔⊔⊔⊔ GREENS: _____

MOVEMENT: _____ ENERGY: _____

PRIORITIES FOR TODAY:

1. _____

2. _____

TODAY I LET GO OF: _____

_____

_____

_____

_____

_____

_____

ONE DREAM I AM WORKING ON: _____

_____

_____

_____

_____

_____

_____

"My body is beautiful and strong. I celebrate my body today."

DATE_____

SLEEP: ☐ 3-5hours ☐ 5-6hours ☐ 7+hours

WATER: ⬛⬛⬛⬛⬛⬛⬛ GREENS: _____

MOVEMENT: _____ ENERGY: _____

PRIORITIES FOR TODAY:

1. _____

2. _____

TODAY I AM GRATEFUL FOR:

1. _____

_____

2. _____

_____

3. _____

_____

AFFIRMATION: _____

_____

_____

_____

_____

_____

_____

_____

_____

"This is a wonderful day. I've never seen this one before." —Unknown

DATE_____

SLEEP: ☐ 3-5hours ☐ 5-6hours ☐ 7+hours

WATER: ⊔ ⊔ ⊔ ⊔ ⊔ ⊔ ⊔ ⊔ GREENS: _____

MOVEMENT: _____ ENERGY: _____

PRIORITIES FOR TODAY:

1. _____

2. _____

MY WINS:

1. _____

_____

2. _____

_____

3. _____

_____

WHERE CAN I SAVE ENERGY TODAY? _____

_____

_____

_____

_____

_____

_____

_____

"I celebrate my individuality. No one is quite like me."

DATE_____

SLEEP: ☐ 3-5hours ☐ 5-6hours ☐ 7+hours

WATER: ☐☐☐☐☐☐☐ GREENS: _____

MOVEMENT: _____ ENERGY: _____

PRIORITIES FOR TODAY:

1. _____

2. _____

I FELT MY BEST TODAY WHEN: _____

_____

_____

_____

_____

_____

_____

_____

ONE GOAL I AM WORKING ON:_____

_____

_____

_____

_____

_____

_____

_____

"Success is only meaningful and enjoyable if it feels like your own."
—Michelle Obama

DATE_____

SLEEP: ☐ 3-5hours ☐ 5-6hours ☐ 7+hours

WATER: ☐☐☐☐☐☐☐ GREENS: _____

MOVEMENT: _____ ENERGY: _____

PRIORITIES FOR TODAY:

1. _____

2. _____

TODAY I SMILED BECAUSE: _____

_____

_____

_____

_____

_____

_____

_____

ONE HARD THING I DID TODAY (OR YESTERDAY): _____

_____

_____

_____

_____

_____

_____

_____

"I believe in myself. I am worthy."

DATE_____

SLEEP: ☐ 3-5hours ☐ 5-6hours ☐ 7+hours

WATER: ⊔ ⊔ ⊔ ⊔ ⊔ ⊔ ⊔ GREENS: _____

MOVEMENT: _____ ENERGY: _____

PRIORITIES FOR TODAY:

1. _____

2. _____

TODAY I LET GO OF: _____

_____

_____

_____

_____

_____

_____

ONE DREAM I AM WORKING ON: _____

_____

_____

_____

_____

_____

_____

"I've learned that people will forget what you said, people will forget what you did, but they will never forget how you made them feel." —Maya Angelou

DATE_____

SLEEP: ☐ 3-5hours ☐ 5-6hours ☐ 7+hours

WATER: ☐☐☐☐☐☐☐☐ GREENS: _____

MOVEMENT: _____ ENERGY: _____

PRIORITIES FOR TODAY:

1. _____

2. _____

TODAY I AM GRATEFUL FOR:

1. _____

_____

2. _____

_____

3. _____

_____

AFFIRMATION: _____

_____

_____

_____

_____

_____

_____

_____

"I am safe. I feel peace. I feel loved."

I want you to envision your life like a staircase. Each step of that staircase represents something we do for ourselves. The goal is to never ever reach the top, the goal is to just always keep climbing. Living your life with inner peace and contentment is the most incredible accomplishment and that takes continual effort. One step each day or each week or each month or whatever timeline works for you, we will keep protecting our peace and contentment by climbing the stairs. The following pages each represent a step in that staircase.

Write down your biggest dream for your life. It doesn't matter how out there it may seem, just let your pen go. Include as many little details as you can, especially the ones that make your heart feel full. When you are done, close your eyes and spend five minutes envisioning that this dream is real and you are living it right now. Revisit this dream as often as you can. Shifting your energy to this feel good space will help you attract more of that into your life. You can do anything you set your mind on, so set your mind on good stuff. Go big!!!!!

_____

_____

_____

_____

_____

_____

_____

_____

_____

_____

_____

_____

_____

_____

_____

_____

"What you seek is seeking you." —Rumi

"One who conquers the sea today is ready to conquer the ocean tomorrow."
—Matshona Dhliwayo

Create a power statement for yourself. Write down the things that you love about yourself. If that feels too big, write down the things you like about yourself and you will work on loving them. Even if in writing it you have a hard time believing it, do it anyway. I want you to write as much as you can, write about the things you are good at, your kindness, the love you give people and the impact you being you makes on the world. If you are struggling with this, think about what a friend or family member would write for you. Come back and reread this often.

Ex: "I am a warrior. I am strong. I am brave"

_____
_____
_____
_____
_____
_____
_____
_____
_____
_____
_____
_____
_____
_____
_____
_____

"There is no education like adversity." —Benjamin Disraeli

"I believe in the power of my soul."

Find a picture of yourself as a little girl or boy. Write this child an "I'm proud of you for" letter with the kindness that you would actually deliver if you two could have a conversation. Now look at yourself in the mirror and reread this letter to your present self. He/She is a beautiful soul who deserves a beautiful life.

_____

_____

_____

_____

_____

_____

_____

_____

_____

_____

_____

_____

_____

_____

_____

_____

_____

_____

_____

"Alone we can do so little, together we can do so much." —Helen Keller

"I am so proud of my journey."

Make a list of your limiting beliefs. What gets in your way? What are the things you tell yourself that you can't do? When you are done, reflect on where you think these things come from? Take your time on this and write it down. Was it something that happened when you were younger? Was it something someone told you that you couldn't do, or you weren't good at?

When you are done, repeat this statement with each thing on your list "I release this limiting belief that no longer serves me. I choose differently now. I am capable of anything I set my mind on and I believe in myself."

Cross out each limiting belief after you have repeated this statement or you can even tear our this page and rip it up. :) This is a big step in the staircase and it's ok if you have to climb it a few times. This is a big one. You are awesome!

_____

_____

_____

_____

_____

_____

_____

_____

_____

_____

_____

_____

"I am the dreamer of my dreams."

"I have not failed. I've just found 10,000 ways that won't work."
—Thomas Edison

Make a list of the things that make you the happiest in life. It doesn't matter if you haven't done some of these things in a long time, just write down anything that lights you up or once lit you up in your life (I'm sure it still does). Pick one of these things and schedule time in the next 7 days to do it. Come back and write it down when it's done. Pick a set amount of time that works for you and complete everything you wrote down on this list. Each time you check something off, come back and write it down. We live better when we follow our passions. You've got this!

_____

_____

_____

_____

_____

_____

_____

_____

_____

_____

_____

_____

_____

_____

_____

_____

"I love who I am becoming."

_____

_____

_____

_____

_____

_____

_____

_____

_____

_____

_____

_____

_____

_____

_____

_____

_____

_____

_____

_____

_____

_____

_____

_____

_____

_____

_____

_____

*"I will not let anyone walk through my mind
with their dirty feet."* —Mahatma Gandhi

What is one thing you have dreamed about or always wanted to try but always found a reason not to do? It can be anything - big or small. Run a 5km, sky dive, take a pottery class, start a business, go sailing, e transfers, tik tok haha, it can literally be anything...Pick something, write it down and give yourself a realistic timeline to get it done. If it's something that can be done today or this week- let's go! If it's something like a big trip or training for a marathon, set the stage by signing up or picking a date and get started. Come back and update your progress here.

_____

_____

_____

_____

_____

_____

_____

_____

_____

_____

_____

_____

_____

_____

_____

_____

"I move my body to cleanse my soul."

"I am worthy of living out my wildest dreams."

What is bravery to you? Not Braveheart bravery but real life, everyday bravery. Who is someone in your life that has been a true example of bravery. Write down why this person inspires or has inspired you. Make a copy of this and send it to this person. If they are no longer with you, take comfort in reading it aloud. They know.

_____

_____

_____

_____

_____

_____

_____

_____

_____

_____

_____

_____

_____

_____

_____

_____

_____

_____

_____

_____

"I have a beautiful heart. My light is needed in the world."

_____

_____

_____

_____

_____

_____

_____

_____

_____

_____

_____

_____

_____

_____

_____

_____

_____

_____

_____

_____

_____

_____

_____

_____

_____

_____

_____

"You have to sniff out joy. Keep your nose to the joy trail."

Write down a time in your life that you had to be brave. This is something we don't recognize enough. When is a time in your life that you have been through something hard and you kept going and you made it through. This is so important. You are so strong and sometimes you just forget how much. One of my favourite quotes is "you never know how strong you can be until being strong is the only choice you have." Unknown. Today acknowledge that unknown strength in you.

_____
_____
_____
_____
_____
_____
_____
_____
_____
_____
_____
_____
_____
_____
_____
_____
_____
_____

"In a world where you can be anything, be kind." —Unknown

"There's a way to do it better. Find it." —Thomas Edison

Write down something you have done in your life that you are really proud of. Give lots of details and don't hold back. It can be a school project that you did 30 years ago that you poured your heart into, it can be the children you made, the career you have built or getting up when your alarm went off when you didn't want to. Just pick one thing and give yourself a personal fist pound/ high five, woohoo because you rock and you are awesome.

_____

_____

_____

_____

_____

_____

_____

_____

_____

_____

_____

_____

_____

_____

_____

_____

_____

"Be truthful, gentle and fearless." —Mahatma Gandhi

"Comparison is the thief of joy." —Eleanor Rosevelt

This one is really important. Ask 5 people to write down something that they love about you. They can write it here or you can copy down what they have written. Make sure you put their name beside it. Reread this every single day and more than that on the days when you need reminders of how beautiful and amazing you are. You can always add to this list. Five is your starting point. I will give you number 1:

"You are such a special person and I'm so glad that you are here. Even if we may have never met, I feel and am touched by your kindness, your compassion and your inner strength. I hope you know how important you are and the light you bring into this world. My hope for you is that you learn to truly appreciate your amazing self, how much happiness you deserve and that you are so truly awesome." —Tracey Gairns Brioux

_____

_____

_____

_____

_____

_____

_____

_____

_____

_____

_____

_____

"I believe in my magic."

_"What you think, you become. What you think, you attract.
What you imagine, you create."_ —Buddha

"As soon as we left the ground I knew I myself had to fly!" —Amelia Earhart